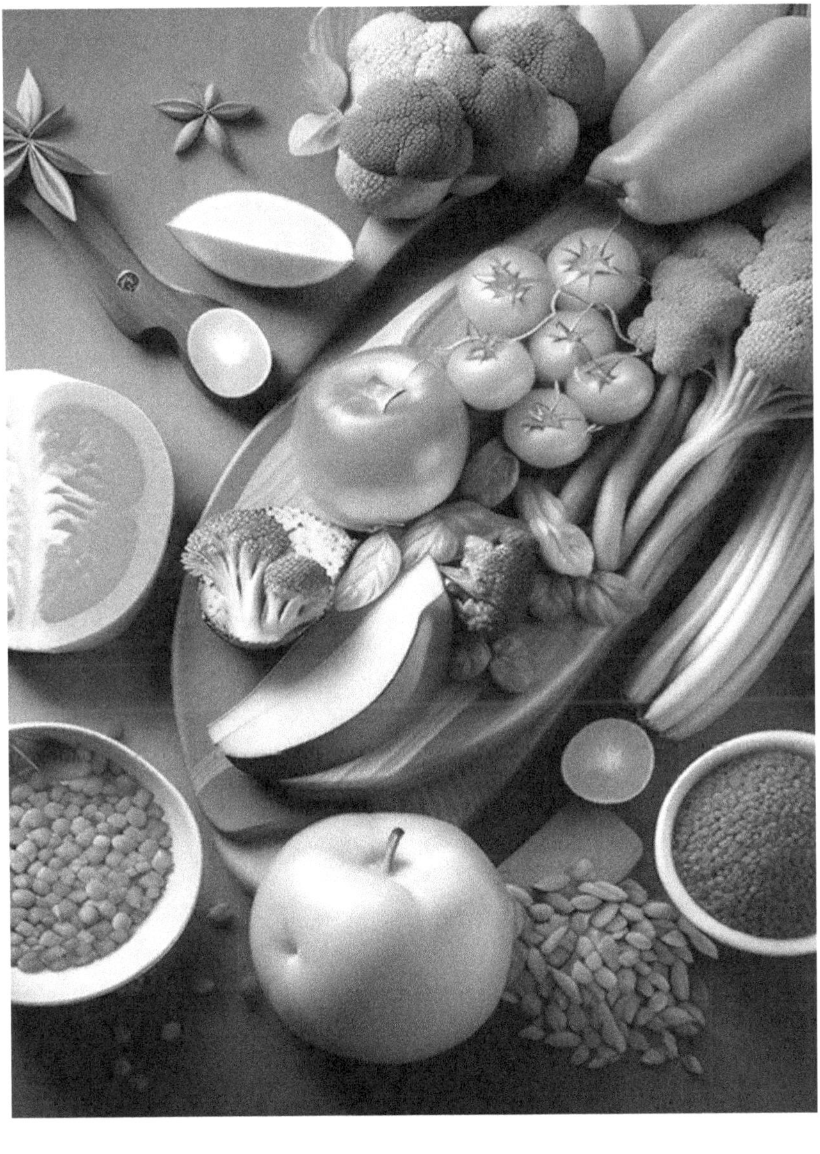

Nourish & Flourish
Unleashing the Power of the Anti-Inflammatory Diet

By

Tommy Blair

Table of Contents

Introduction

Welcome to **"Nourish & Flourish."** In this book, we embark on a transformative journey towards harnessing the incredible potential of an anti-inflammatory diet to enhance our health and well-being.

The human body is a complex and intricate system, and inflammation is a natural response that helps protect and heal us. However, when inflammation becomes chronic and uncontrolled, it can contribute to a wide range of health issues, including arthritis, heart disease, obesity, and even mental health disorders.

Fortunately, we have the power to influence inflammation through the foods we eat. The anti-inflammatory diet is a holistic approach that focuses on consuming foods rich in nutrients, antioxidants, and anti-inflammatory properties while avoiding or minimizing those that promote inflammation.

In this introductory section, we will delve into the inflammatory process, helping you understand how certain foods can either fuel or fight inflammation. We will explore the incredible benefits of adopting an anti-inflammatory diet, from reduced pain and improved digestion to enhanced energy levels and a strengthened immune system.

By embracing the principles of the anti-inflammatory diet, you are taking a proactive step towards optimizing your health and vitality. Throughout this book, we will equip you with the knowledge, practical guidance, and mouthwatering recipes to effortlessly incorporate anti-inflammatory foods into your daily life.

Get ready to nourish your body, balance your immune system, and flourish in radiant health. Let's embark on this empowering journey together and unlock the full potential of the anti-inflammatory diet.

The food we consume plays a significant role in modulating inflammation within our bodies. Certain foods can either promote or reduce inflammation, impacting our overall health and well-being. By understanding the inflammatory process and the role of food, we can make informed choices to support an anti-inflammatory lifestyle. Let's delve into the details of the inflammatory process and how food influences it.

Inflammation: The Body's Defense Mechanism
- An essential process that helps protect and heal the body
- Initiated in response to injury, infection, or tissue damage
- Involves the release of various chemical mediators and immune cells

Chronic Inflammation: The Culprit of Disease
- Prolonged and persistent inflammation
- Associated with a range of chronic diseases, including cardiovascular disease, diabetes, and autoimmune disorders

- Can be influenced by dietary factors

Pro-Inflammatory Foods
- Foods that promote inflammation within the body
- High in refined sugars and carbohydrates
- Processed and fried foods include saturated and trans fats.
- Excessive consumption of red and processed meats
- Artificial additives and preservatives in packaged and processed foods

Anti-Inflammatory Foods
- Foods that help reduce inflammation and promote overall health
- Rich in antioxidants, phytochemicals, and omega-3 fatty acids
- Vegetables and Fruits, especially those with vibrant colors
- Healthy fats, including those found in fatty fish, nuts, seeds, and olive oil
- Whole grains, legumes, and fiber-rich foods
- Herbs and spices with anti-inflammatory properties

The Gut Microbiome and Inflammation

- The complex ecosystem of microorganisms residing in our digestive system
- Plays an important role in immunological function and inflammatory control.
- Certain foods can influence the composition and diversity of the gut microbiome, impacting inflammation levels

Individual Variations and Sensitivities

- People may react differently to certain foods
- Food sensitivities or allergies can trigger an inflammatory response
- Identifying and eliminating specific trigger foods can help reduce inflammation

The Power of an Anti-Inflammatory Diet

- Adopting an anti-inflammatory diet can help manage and reduce chronic inflammation

- Promotes overall health, cardiovascular health, and a balanced immune system
- Supports optimal gut health and a diverse gut microbiome

By understanding the inflammatory process and the impact of food choices, we can make informed decisions to support our body's natural healing mechanisms and reduce chronic inflammation. Embracing an anti-inflammatory diet rich in whole, unprocessed foods and avoiding pro-inflammatory foods can contribute to a healthier, more vibrant life. Let's harness the power of food to nourish our bodies and promote well-being.

Benefits of an Anti-Inflammatory Diet

Adopting an anti-inflammatory diet can bring about numerous benefits for our overall health and well-being. By reducing chronic inflammation, we can positively impact various systems within our bodies, leading to improved physical and mental health. Let's explore the wide-ranging benefits of embracing an anti-inflammatory diet.

Reduced Risk of Chronic Diseases

- Reducing a person's chance of developing cardiovascular disorders, such as heart disease and stroke
- Decreasing the likelihood of developing chronic conditions like diabetes, obesity, and metabolic syndrome
- Protecting against certain types of cancer, such as colorectal and breast cancer

Enhanced Immune Function
- Supporting a healthy immune response and strengthening the body's defense against infections and diseases
- Promoting optimal function of immune cells and reducing excessive immune activation
- Lowering the risk of autoimmune disorders by modulating immune system activity

Improved Digestive Health
- Alleviating symptoms of inflammatory bowel diseases, such as Crohn's disease and ulcerative colitis
- Soothing gastrointestinal inflammation and promoting gut health

- Enhancing nutrient absorption and optimizing digestion

Joint Health and Pain Reduction

- Easing symptoms of arthritis and other inflammatory joint conditions
- Reducing joint pain, stiffness, and swelling
- Supporting joint mobility and overall musculoskeletal health

Balanced Mood and Mental Well-being

- Mitigating inflammation's impact on mental health conditions, such as depression and anxiety
- Supporting brain health and cognitive function
- Promoting a balanced mood and emotional well-being

Weight Management

- Facilitating healthy weight loss and weight maintenance
- Reducing adipose tissue inflammation and metabolic dysfunction

- Promoting a healthier body composition and improved metabolic profile

Enhanced Energy Levels and Vitality
- Combating fatigue and boosting overall energy levels
- Improving sleep quality and promoting restorative rest
- Enhancing physical performance and endurance

By embracing an anti-inflammatory diet, we empower ourselves to optimize our health and enjoy a higher quality of life. The wide-ranging benefits extend beyond just reducing inflammation, positively influencing various body systems, and promoting overall well-being. So, let's embark on this journey towards better health and unlock the full potential of the anti-inflammatory diet.

Chapter 1

Anti-Inflammatory Foods

Incorporating anti-inflammatory foods into your diet is a key component of the anti-inflammatory lifestyle. These nourishing and healing foods possess powerful properties that can help reduce inflammation, support optimal health, and boost your overall well-being. Let's explore a variety of anti-inflammatory foods and learn how to include them in your daily meals.

Fruits and Vegetables

- Berries: Blueberries, strawberries, raspberries, and more
- Leafy greens: Collard greens, Spinach, kale, and Swiss chard,
- Cruciferous vegetables: Cauliflower, Broccoli, cabbage, and Brussels sprouts
- Bright-colored vegetables: Bell peppers, tomatoes, carrots, and sweet potatoes
- Citrus fruits: Oranges, lemons, grapefruits, and limes

Healthy Fats

- Omega-3 fatty acids: Fatty fish (salmon, sardines), flaxseeds, chia seeds, and walnuts
- Extra virgin olive oil
- Avocado and avocado oil

Lean Proteins

- Fatty fish: Salmon, mackerel, trout, and herring
- Skinless poultry: Chicken and turkey breast
- Legumes: Kidney beans, chickpeas, black beans, and lentils
- Nuts and seeds: Almonds, walnuts, pumpkin seeds, and chia seeds
- Tofu and tempeh

Whole Grains

- Quinoa
- Brown rice
- Oats
- Whole wheat products (bread, pasta)

Herbs and Spices

- Turmeric
- Ginger
- Garlic
- Cinnamon
- Rosemary
- Basil
- Oregano
- Cayenne pepper

Green Tea

- Sencha
- Gyokuro
- Kabusecha
- Matcha
- Tencha
- Genmaicha
- Hojicha

Probiotic Foods

- Yogurt (unsweetened and probiotic-rich)
- Kefir
- Sauerkraut
- Kimchi

By incorporating these anti-inflammatory foods into your meals and snacks, you can harness their healing power and support your body in combating inflammation. Remember to prioritize a diverse and balanced diet, focusing on whole, unprocessed foods for optimal benefits. Let's explore delicious recipes and creative ways to enjoy these anti-inflammatory foods as we embark on our journey towards improved health and vitality.

The Power of Plant-Based Foods

Plant-based foods are a cornerstone of the anti-inflammatory diet, providing a wealth of nutrients, antioxidants, and phytochemicals that can help reduce inflammation and promote optimal health. Embracing the power of plant-based foods not only supports your well-being but also contributes to environmental sustainability. Let's explore the incredible benefits and diverse range of plant-based foods you can incorporate into your anti-inflammatory diet.

Nutrient-Rich Fruits and Vegetables

- Abundance of vitamins, minerals, and fiber
- High antioxidant content to combat oxidative stress

- Colorful varieties for maximum nutritional benefits

Leafy Greens and Cruciferous Vegetables
- Dark leafy greens (spinach, kale, Swiss chard) packed with vitamins and minerals
- Cruciferous vegetables (broccoli, cauliflower, Brussels sprouts) containing sulforaphane and other anti-inflammatory compounds

Colorful Berries
- Rich in antioxidants, including anthocyanins
- Blueberries, strawberries, raspberries, and blackberries

Healthy Fats from Plants
- Avocado and avocado oil for monounsaturated fats
- Nuts and seeds (almonds, walnuts, flaxseeds) for omega-3 fatty acids and antioxidants

Legumes and Pulses

- Excellent sources of plant-based protein and fiber
- Lentils, chickpeas, black beans, and kidney beans

Whole Grains and Ancient Grains

- Fiber-rich options for sustained energy and gut health
- Brown rice, quinoa, oats, and whole wheat products

Plant-Based Protein Sources

- Tofu and tempeh for soy-based protein
- Plant-based protein powders (pea, hemp, rice)

Herbs and Spices

- Turmeric, ginger, garlic, and cinnamon for their potent anti-inflammatory properties
- Rosemary, basil, oregano, and cayenne pepper for flavor and health benefits

Herbal Teas

- Chamomile, peppermint, and ginger teas for their soothing and anti-inflammatory effects

By incorporating a variety of plant-based foods into your meals, you can experience the immense benefits they offer in reducing inflammation, supporting healthy weight management, improving digestion, and promoting overall vitality. Remember to prioritize organic and locally sourced options whenever possible to maximize nutritional value and minimize exposure to pesticides. Let's embrace the power of plant-based foods and embark on a journey of vibrant health and well-being.

Incorporating Healthy Fats and Proteins

Healthy fats and proteins are essential components of an anti-inflammatory diet. They provide necessary nutrients, promote satiety, and play a crucial role in reducing inflammation and supporting overall health. Let's explore various sources of healthy fats and proteins that you can incorporate into your meals.

Fatty Fish

- Salmon, mackerel, sardines, and trout
- Omega-3 fatty acids, which have potent anti-inflammatory properties in abundant
- Grilled, baked, or pan-seared preparations

Plant-Based Omega-3 Sources
- Flaxseeds, chia seeds, and hemp seeds
- Walnuts and almonds
- Incorporate into smoothies, salads, or sprinkle over dishes

Avocado and Avocado Oil
- Creamy and nutrient-dense fruit
- Avocado oil for cooking and salad dressings
- Spread avocado on toast, add to salads, or use as a replacement for unhealthy fats

Nuts and Seeds
- Almonds, walnuts, pistachios, pumpkin seeds, and sunflower seeds
- Rich in healthy fats, protein, and fiber
- Enjoy as a snack, sprinkle on salads or yogurt, or use in homemade granola and energy bars

Legumes and Pulses

- Lentils, chickpeas, black beans, and kidney beans
- Excellent plant-based protein sources
- Use in soups, stews, salads, or as a base for veggie burgers and dips

Tofu and Tempeh

- Soy-based protein options
- Versatile and absorb flavors well in various dishes
- Stir-fry, grill, bake, or use in curries and stir-fries

Greek Yogurt and Cottage Cheese

- High-protein dairy options
- Choose plain, unsweetened varieties for maximum health benefits
- Enjoy as a snack, add to smoothies, or use as a creamy topping for dishes

Eggs

- Excellent source of protein and essential nutrients
- Opt for organic or free-range eggs whenever possible

- Incorporate into omelets, scrambles, or use for baking and cooking

By incorporating these healthy fats and protein sources into your meals, you can promote satiety, support muscle repair and growth, and reduce inflammation. Remember to prioritize quality and balance in your dietary choices, and opt for organic and sustainable options whenever possible. Let's embrace these nourishing ingredients and create delicious, anti-inflammatory meals that support our overall well-being.

The Best Anti-Inflammatory Herbs and Spices

Herbs and spices not only add delightful flavors to our meals but also offer powerful anti-inflammatory properties. Incorporating these natural ingredients into your cooking can enhance the taste of your dishes while providing numerous health benefits. Let's explore some of the best anti-inflammatory herbs and spices you can incorporate into your culinary creations.

Turmeric

- The active compound in turmeric which exhibits potent anti-inflammatory properties is curcumin
- Enhances the flavor of curries, soups, and stir-fries
- Combine with black pepper to enhance curcumin absorption

Ginger

- Contains gingerol, a powerful anti-inflammatory compound
- Gives meals a spicy and toasty taste.
- Use in stir-fries, sauces, marinades, and teas

Garlic

- Allicin, a sulfur compound in garlic, provides anti-inflammatory benefits
- Elevates the flavor of savory dishes
- Add to sautés, roasted vegetables, sauces, and dressings

Cinnamon

- Contains antioxidants and anti-inflammatory compounds
- Offers a sweet and warm flavor

- Sprinkle on oatmeal, yogurt, smoothies, and baked goods

Rosemary

- Contains rosmarinic acid, which has anti-inflammatory effects
- Imparts a fragrant and savory taste
- Use in roasted vegetables, grilled meats, marinades, and dressings

Basil

- Rich in antioxidants and anti-inflammatory compounds
- Adds a fresh and aromatic flavor to dishes
- Incorporate in pesto, salads, sauces, and pasta dishes

Oregano

- Contains the compound carvacrol, which has anti-inflammatory properties
- Offers a robust and slightly bitter taste
- Use in Italian dishes, marinades, and tomato-based sauces

Cayenne Pepper

- Capsaicin in cayenne pepper has anti-inflammatory effects
- Provides a spicy kick to meals
- Add to soups, stews, chili, and roasted vegetables

Incorporating these herbs and spices into your cooking not only enhances the taste of your meals but also provides a natural way to reduce inflammation in the body. Experiment with different combinations and find ways to incorporate these ingredients into your favorite recipes. Let the flavors and health benefits of these anti-inflammatory herbs and spices elevate your culinary experience and promote your well-being.

Chapter 2

Foods to Avoid

To maintain an anti-inflammatory diet and reduce the risk of chronic inflammation, it is essential to be mindful of certain foods that can promote inflammation within the body. By minimizing or avoiding these foods, you can support your overall health and well-being. Let's explore the key foods to avoid in an anti-inflammatory diet.

Refined Sugars and Sweetened Beverages
- Soda, fruit juices with added sugars, energy drinks
- Candy, pastries, cookies, and other sugary treats
- Excessive consumption of sugar can lead to inflammation and increased health risks

Trans Fats and Processed Fats
- Fried foods: French fries, fried chicken, and other deep-fried items

- Processed snacks: Chips, crackers, and packaged baked goods
- Margarine and vegetable shortening
- Trans fats increase inflammation and raise the risk of heart disease and other health problems

Red and Processed Meats

- Beef, pork, lamb, and processed meats (hot dogs, sausages, deli meats)
- High in saturated fats and potentially harmful compounds
- Linked to increased inflammation and various health conditions

Highly Processed Foods

- Packaged snacks: Chips, pretzels, and other processed snacks
- Instant meals: Frozen pizzas, microwavable dinners, and processed convenience foods
- Foods containing artificial additives, preservatives, and refined grains
- These foods often lack nutrients and can contribute to inflammation and poor health outcomes

Vegetable Oils and Hydrogenated Oils
- Canola, soybean, corn, and sunflower oils
- Hydrogenated oils, found in many processed foods
- These oils are high in omega-6 fatty acids, which can promote inflammation when consumed in excess

Excessive Alcohol Consumption
- Heavy and regular alcohol consumption can trigger inflammation
- Moderation is key, and excessive intake should be avoided

Additives and Artificial Sweeteners
- Artificial sweeteners: Aspartame, sucralose, saccharin, and others
- Food additives: MSG (monosodium glutamate), artificial colors, and flavors
- These additives may cause inflammation in certain individuals

Gluten and Wheat (for those with sensitivities)
- Gluten-containing grains: wheat, barley, and rye

- Some individuals may have gluten sensitivity or celiac disease, leading to inflammation and digestive issues

By being mindful of these foods and making healthier alternatives, you can reduce inflammation and support your overall well-being. Focus on consuming whole, unprocessed foods, and opt for cooking methods such as grilling, baking, steaming, or sautéing instead of deep frying. Let's make informed choices about the foods we consume and prioritize a nourishing and anti-inflammatory diet.

Inflammatory Foods to Eliminate

Eliminating or minimizing certain inflammatory foods from your diet is crucial to support an anti-inflammatory lifestyle and reduce chronic inflammation. By avoiding these foods, you can promote optimal health and well-being. Let's explore the key inflammatory foods that you should consider eliminating.

Processed and Refined Grains
- White bread, white rice, and refined pasta

- Processed breakfast cereals and baked goods made with refined flour
- These foods can lead to inflammation and spikes in blood sugar levels

Artificial Trans Fats

- Partially hydrogenated oils found in processed foods and margarine
- Deep-fried foods, including French fries and doughnuts
- Trans fats increase inflammation and raise the risk of heart disease and other health issues

Sugary and Sweetened Beverages

- Soda, fruit juices with added sugars, energy drinks, and sweetened tea/coffee
- High-fructose corn syrup and other artificial sweeteners
- These beverages contribute to inflammation and can lead to weight gain and chronic diseases

Processed Meats

- Hot dogs, sausages, bacon, and deli meats

- These meats contain preservatives, additives, and high levels of sodium, leading to inflammation and increased health risks

Saturated and Trans Fats
- Fatty cuts of red meat, full-fat dairy products, and butter
- Processed snacks and baked goods with high levels of saturated fats
- These fats can increase inflammation and raise the risk of heart disease and other health problems

High-Fructose Corn Syrup and Added Sugars
- Found in many processed foods, including condiments, sauces, and sweetened beverages
- These added sugars contribute to inflammation, weight gain, and various chronic diseases

Artificial Food Additives
- Artificial colors, flavors, and preservatives found in processed foods

- MSG (monosodium glutamate) and other flavor enhancers
- These additives can trigger inflammation in certain individuals

Excessive Alcohol Consumption
- Heavy and regular alcohol consumption can lead to inflammation and damage various organs
- Limit alcohol intake and practice moderation for overall health benefits

By eliminating or significantly reducing these inflammatory foods from your diet, you can reduce inflammation, support a healthy immune system, and lower the risk of chronic diseases. Instead, focus on consuming whole, unprocessed foods, including plenty of fruits, vegetables, lean proteins, and healthy fats. Let's make conscious choices about the foods we consume and prioritize an anti-inflammatory diet for our well-being.

Hidden Inflammatory Culprits

In addition to the obvious inflammatory foods, there are several hidden culprits that can contribute to inflammation within the body. These culprits may go unnoticed but can have a significant impact on your overall health and well-being. By being aware of these hidden inflammatory triggers, you can make informed choices to reduce inflammation and support an anti-inflammatory lifestyle. Let's uncover some of the hidden inflammatory culprits.

Vegetable Oils and Omega-6 Fatty Acids

- Despite the fact that omega-6 fatty acids are essential, inflammation can be exacerbated due to an imbalance between omega-6 and omega-3 fatty acids.
- Excessive consumption of vegetable oils high in omega-6 fatty acids, such as soybean oil, corn oil, and sunflower oil
- Opt for healthier alternatives like olive oil, avocado oil, or coconut oil in moderation

Processed and Packaged Foods

- Many processed and packaged foods contain hidden inflammatory ingredients
- Artificial additives, preservatives, and flavor enhancers like MSG (monosodium glutamate)

- Read ingredient labels carefully and choose whole, unprocessed options whenever possible

Gluten (for those with sensitivities)
- Wheat, rye, and barley all contain the protein known as gluten.
- Some individuals may have gluten sensitivities or celiac disease, leading to inflammation and digestive issues
- If you suspect gluten intolerance, consider eliminating gluten-containing foods or consult with a healthcare professional for a proper diagnosis

Artificial Sweeteners
- Artificial sweeteners like aspartame, sucralose, and saccharin
- While they offer low-calorie alternatives to sugar, some studies suggest they may contribute to inflammation and negatively impact gut health
- Limit or avoid artificial sweeteners and opt for natural sweeteners like stevia or moderate consumption of natural sugars

Dairy Products (for those with lactose intolerance or sensitivities)

- Some individuals could have a dairy sensitivity or lactose intolerance.
- Dairy can lead to digestive issues, inflammation, and other symptoms in sensitive individuals
- Experiment with dairy alternatives like almond milk, coconut milk, or lactose-free dairy products if needed

Hidden Food Allergies or Sensitivities

- Some individuals may have hidden food allergies or sensitivities that can trigger inflammation
- Common allergens include nuts, shellfish, eggs, and soy
- If you suspect a food allergy or sensitivity, consider an elimination diet or seek guidance from a healthcare professional

Excessive Intake of Alcohol and Caffeine

- While moderate alcohol consumption may have some health benefits, excessive

intake can lead to inflammation and other health issues
- Excessive caffeine consumption can also contribute to inflammation and disrupt sleep patterns
- Moderation is key when consuming alcohol and caffeine-containing beverages

By being mindful of these hidden inflammatory culprits, you can make informed choices to reduce inflammation and support your overall health. Listen to your body, experiment with different foods, and consult with healthcare professionals when needed to identify any hidden triggers that may be causing inflammation. Let's uncover and eliminate these hidden culprits to embrace an anti-inflammatory lifestyle.

Chapter 3

The Anti-Inflammatory Meal Plan

Following an anti-inflammatory meal plan can help you reduce inflammation, support your overall health, and promote well-being. By incorporating a variety of nutrient-dense foods and avoiding inflammatory triggers, you can create a balanced and delicious meal plan that nourishes your body. Let's explore a sample anti-inflammatory meal plan to get you started.

Note: *For informative reasons only, use this meal plan. It is essential to tailor the plan to your specific dietary needs, preferences, and any underlying health conditions. For individualized guidance, speak with a registered dietitian or healthcare professional.*

Day 1:
- **Breakfast:** Mushroom omelet and spinach with avocado slices
- **Snack:** Carrot sticks with hummus

- **Lunch:** Quinoa and roasted asparagus with grilled salmon
- **Snack:** Mixed berries with a handful of almonds
- **Dinner:** Brown rice and steamed broccoli with baked chicken breast
- **Dessert:** Greek yogurt with a drizzle of honey and sprinkled with cinnamon

Day 2:

- **Breakfast:** Overnight chia seed pudding topped with fresh berries and crushed walnuts
- **Snack:** Sliced cucumbers with tahini dip
- **Lunch:** Grilled chicken, cherry tomatoes, cucumber, and mixed greens in a quinoa salad.
- **Snack:** Apple slices with almond butter
- **Dinner:** Roasted brussels sprouts and sweet potato wedges with baked cod
- **Dessert:** Baked apples topped with a sprinkle of cinnamon and a dollop of coconut yogurt

Day 3:

- **Breakfast:** Spinach, banana, almond milk, and a scoop of protein powder combined to make a green smoothie.
- **Snack:** Kale chips
- **Lunch:** A side of mixed green salad with lentil soup
- **Snack:** Fresh pineapple chunks
- **Dinner:** Brown rice and grilled tofu stir-fry with a variety of colorful veggies
- **Dessert:** Dark chocolate squares

Day 4:

- **Breakfast:** Veggie scramble with bell peppers, onions, and zucchini
- **Snack:** Edamame beans
- **Lunch:** Roasted chicken breast with quinoa, roasted vegetables, and a side of mixed greens
- **Snack:** Homemade trail mix with almonds, walnuts, dried cranberries, and pumpkin seeds
- **Dinner:** Marinara sauce and zucchini noodles with baked turkey meatballs
- **Dessert:** Berry and coconut milk smoothie

Day 5:

- **Breakfast:** Oatmeal topped with blueberries, sliced banana, and a sprinkle of flaxseeds
- **Snack:** Greek yogurt with almond slices and a honey drizzle
- **Lunch:** Grilled shrimp skewers with quinoa tabbouleh salad
- **Snack:** Celery sticks with almond butter
- **Dinner:** Roasted asparagus and cauliflower rice with baked salmon
- **Dessert:** Mango and coconut chia pudding

Always remember to stay hydrated throughout the day and modify portion sizes to suit your particular requirements. Aim for a colorful and varied plate to ensure you're getting a wide range of nutrients. Incorporate herbs and spices known for their anti-inflammatory properties to add flavor to your meals.

This meal plan provides a starting point for your anti-inflammatory journey. Feel free to modify and experiment with different recipes and ingredients that align with your preferences and dietary needs. Make choices that support your well-being by listening to your body. Enjoy the process of nourishing yourself with delicious and anti-inflammatory foods.

A 7-Day Meal Plan

Here's a 7-day anti-inflammatory meal plan to help you get started:

Day 1:

- **Breakfast:** Banana, kale, spinach, almond milk, and a scoop of protein powder combined to make a green smoothie.
- **Snack:** Carrot sticks with hummus.
- **Lunch:** Grilled chicken breast with mixed greens, cherry tomatoes, cucumber, and a drizzle of olive oil and lemon juice.
- **Snack:** Mixed berries with a handful of walnuts.
- **Dinner:** Baked salmon with quinoa and roasted brussels sprouts.
- **Dessert:** Greek yogurt with a sprinkle of cinnamon and sliced almonds.

Day 2:

- **Breakfast:** Quinoa porridge topped with fresh berries, a dollop of almond butter, and a sprinkle of chia seeds.
- **Snack:** Sliced bell peppers with guacamole.
- **Lunch:** Lentil and vegetable soup with a side salad.
- **Snack:** Apple slices with a small handful of cashews.
- **Dinner:** Grilled tofu with stir-fried veggies and brown rice.
- **Dessert:** Dark chocolate squares.

Day 3:

- **Breakfast:** Scrambled eggs with sautéed spinach, tomatoes, and a slice of whole-grain toast.
- **Snack:** Greek yogurt with peach slices and honey drizzle.
- **Lunch:** Quinoa salad with roasted veggies, chickpeas, and a lemon-tahini dressing.
- **Snack:** Celery sticks with almond butter.
- **Dinner:** Baked chicken breast with roasted sweet potatoes and steamed broccoli.

- **Dessert:** Berry and coconut milk smoothie.

Day 4:

- **Breakfast:** Overnight oats made with almond milk, chia seeds, sliced banana, and a sprinkle of cinnamon.
- **Snack:** Edamame beans.
- **Lunch:** Grilled shrimp skewers with quinoa tabbouleh salad.
- **Snack:** Trail mix with almonds, walnuts, dried cranberries, and pumpkin seeds.
- **Dinner:** Baked cod with quinoa and roasted asparagus.
- **Dessert:** Baked apples topped with a sprinkle of nutmeg and a dollop of coconut yogurt.

Day 5:

- **Breakfast:** Veggie scramble with bell peppers, onions, zucchini, and a side of sliced avocado.
- **Snack:** Kale chips.
- **Lunch:** Mixed green salad with grilled chicken, cherry tomatoes, cucumber, and a lemon vinaigrette.

- **Snack:** Fresh pineapple chunks.
- **Dinner:** Baked turkey meatballs with marinara sauce and zucchini noodles.
- **Dessert:** Mango and coconut chia pudding.

Day 6:

- **Breakfast:** Spinach and mushroom omelet with a side of sliced tomatoes.
- **Snack:** Cucumber slices with tzatziki dip.
- **Lunch:** With a side salad and quinoa-stuffed bell peppers.
- **Snack:** Almond milk smoothie with mixed berries and a scoop of protein powder.
- **Dinner:** Grilled salmon with roasted cauliflower and brown rice.
- **Dessert:** Banana "nice" cream made with frozen bananas and topped with crushed almonds.

Day 7:

- **Breakfast:** Avocado toast on whole-grain bread, topped with cherry tomatoes and a sprinkle of hemp seeds.
- **Snack:** Snap peas with hummus.

- **Lunch:** Chickpea and vegetable curry served over brown rice.
- **Snack:** Orange slices with a small handful of pistachios.
- **Dinner:** Baked chicken thighs with roasted root vegetables and quinoa.
- **Dessert:** Chia seed pudding with coconut milk and fresh berries.

If you have specific dietary requirements or preferences, feel free to modify the ingredients and portion sizes. Always remember to stay hydrated by drinking water throughout the day. Enjoy nourishing your body with these delicious and anti-inflammatory meals!

Meal Planning Tips and Tricks

Here are some meal-planning tips and tricks to help you with your anti-inflammatory diet:

- **Plan ahead**

Make time every week to plan your meals. Look for anti-inflammatory recipes and create a meal plan for the upcoming week. On hectic weekdays, this will help you save time and stress.

- **Batch cooking**

Prepare larger portions of meals and divide them into individual servings. This way, you can have ready-made meals for the week, reducing the need for last-minute cooking.

- **Focus on whole foods**

Emphasize whole, unprocessed foods in your meal plan. Include lots of fruits and vegetables, whole grains, lean meats, and healthy fats in your diet. The anti-inflammatory properties of these foods are widely recognized.

- **Variety is key**

Aim to include a variety of colors and flavors in your meals. Different fruits and vegetables provide a range of nutrients and phytochemicals that can help reduce inflammation.

- **Use herbs and spices**

Experiment with herbs and spices that have anti-inflammatory properties, such as turmeric, ginger, garlic, cinnamon, and rosemary. They can add flavor to your dishes while providing additional health benefits.

- **Include omega-3 fatty acids**

Incorporate foods rich in omega-3 fatty acids, such as fatty fish (salmon, mackerel, sardines), walnuts, flaxseeds, and chia seeds. Omega-3s have anti-inflammatory effects and are essential for overall health.

- **Prep in advance**

Take some time to prep ingredients ahead of time. Vegetables should be washed and chopped, grains should be cooked, and proteins should be marinated. This will streamline your cooking process and make it easier to put meals together.

- **Make use of leftovers**

Don't let leftovers go to waste. Plan to have leftover meals for lunches or repurpose them into new dishes. For example, roasted chicken can be used in salads or sandwiches the next day.

- **Snack smart**

Plan for healthy snacks that are anti-inflammatory, such as raw nuts, seeds, fresh fruits, vegetable sticks with hummus, or Greek yogurt with berries.

- **Listen to your body**

Take note of how different meals make you feel. Every person's body may react differently to certain foods, even those generally considered anti-inflammatory. Customize your meal plan based on your body's needs and any specific dietary restrictions or sensitivities you have.

Remember, consistency is key when it comes to an anti-inflammatory diet. Gradually incorporate these tips into your routine and make adjustments as needed. Enjoy the process of nourishing your body with delicious, inflammation-fighting meals!

Chapter 4

Anti-Inflammatory Recipes

To get you started, here are a few anti-inflammatory recipes:

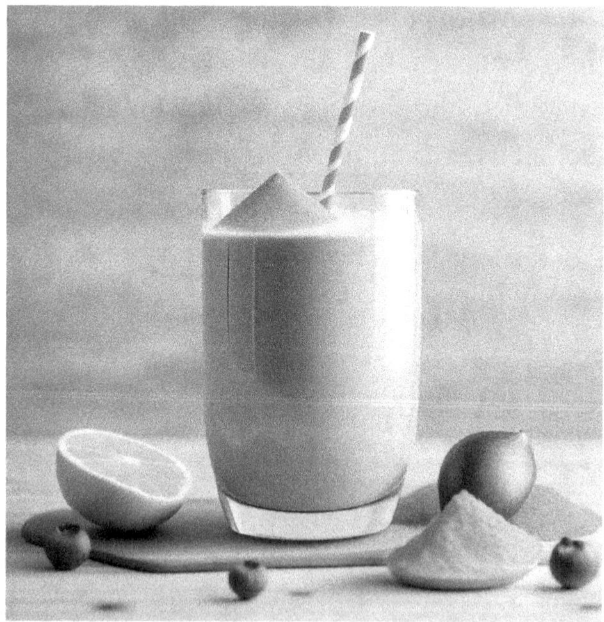

Turmeric Ginger Smoothie

Turmeric Ginger Smoothie:

Ingredients:

- A single cup of almond milk (or any other plant-based milk)
- 1 frozen banana
- 1/2 tsp turmeric powder
- 1/2 tsp grated fresh ginger
- 1 tbsp chia seeds
- 1 teaspoon maple syrup or honey (optional for sweetness)

Instructions:

- All the ingredients should be blended in a blender until smooth.
- Pour into a glass and enjoy this refreshing and anti-inflammatory smoothie.

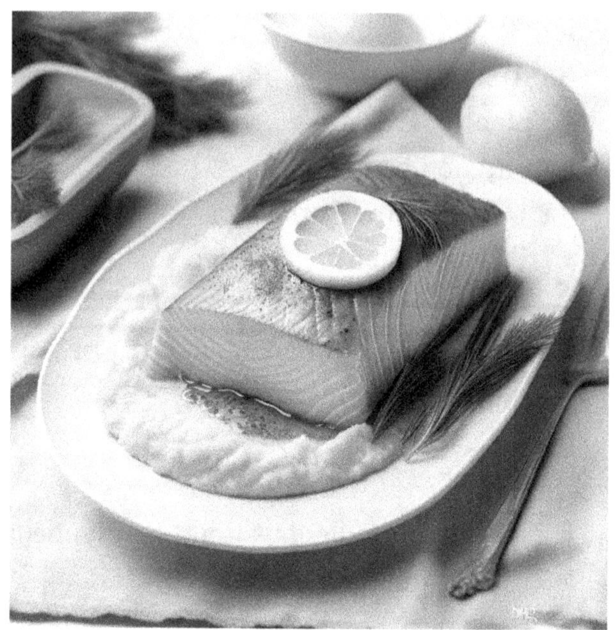

Baked Salmon with Lemon and Dill

Baked Salmon with Lemon and Dill:

Ingredients:

- 2 salmon fillets
- 1 lemon juice
- 2 tbsp chopped fresh dill
- Salt and pepper to taste

Instructions:

- Preheat the oven to 400°F (200°C).

- On a baking sheet lined with parchment paper, put the salmon fillets.
- Drizzle the lemon juice over the salmon and sprinkle with fresh dill, salt, and pepper.
- Salmon should be cooked through and flake easily with a fork after baking for about 15-20 minutes.
- Serve with your choice of roasted vegetables or a side salad.

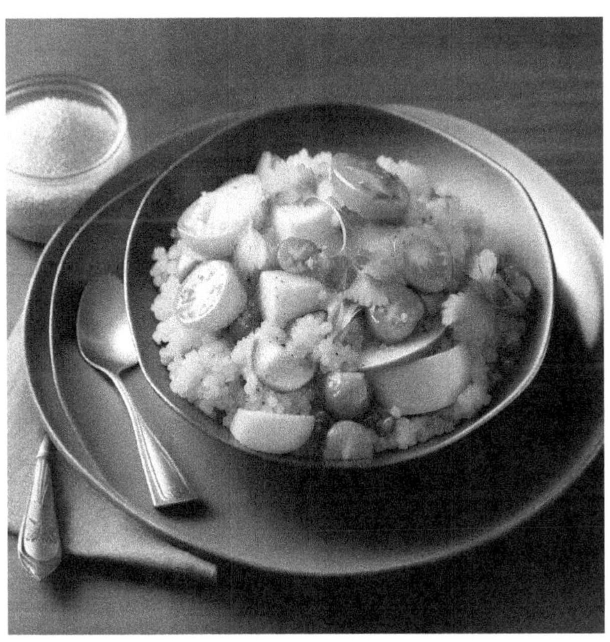

Quinoa Salad with Roasted Vegetables

Ingredients:

- 1 cup cooked quinoa
- 1 cup mixed roasted veggies (such as bell peppers, zucchini, eggplant, and cherry tomatoes)
- 2 cups mixed greens
- 1/4 cup crumbled feta cheese (optional)
- 2 tbsp extra-virgin olive oil
- 1 tbsp balsamic vinegar
- Salt and pepper to taste

Instructions:

- In a large bowl, combine the cooked quinoa, roasted vegetables, mixed greens, and feta cheese.
- To make the dressing, whisk together the olive oil, balsamic vinegar, salt, and pepper in a small bowl.
- To coat, toss the salad with the dressing.
- Serve the salad as a refreshing and nutrient-packed meal.

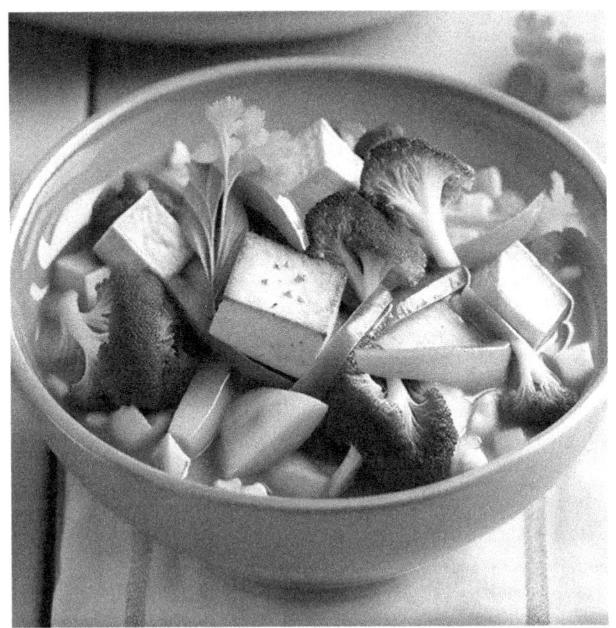

Ginger Garlic Stir-Fried Vegetables with Tofu

Ginger Garlic Stir-Fried Vegetables with Tofu:

Ingredients:

- 1 firm tofu block, drained and cubed
- 2 cups mixed vegetables (such as broccoli, bell peppers, carrots, and snap peas)
- 2 cloves garlic, minced
- 1 tbsp grated fresh ginger
- 2 tbsp low-sodium soy sauce or tamari
- 1 tbsp sesame oil

- 1 tbsp coconut oil (for cooking)

Instructions:

- The coconut oil should be heated over medium-high heat in a large skillet or wok.
- Tofu cubes should be added and cooked until golden brown on all sides. Set aside after removing from the skillet.
- Ginger and garlic should be added to the same skillet. For approximately a minute, stir-fry until fragrant.
- Add the mixed vegetables and cook until crisp-tender.
- Return the tofu to the skillet and drizzle with soy sauce or tamari and sesame oil. Toss to combine.
- Cook for an additional 2-3 minutes until everything is well-coated and heated through.
- Serve the stir-fried vegetables and tofu over brown rice or quinoa for a satisfying meal.

Remember to customize these recipes according to your taste preferences and any specific dietary needs. Enjoy these flavorful and anti-inflammatory dishes as part of your healthy eating plan!

Breakfasts that Fuel Your Day

Here are a few breakfast ideas that will help fuel your day with energy and nutrients:

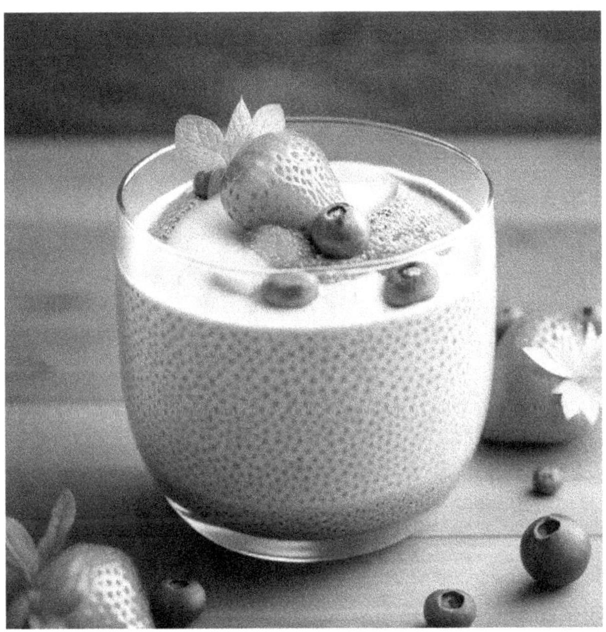

<u>Overnight Chia Pudding</u>

Overnight Chia Pudding:

Ingredients:

- 2 tbsp chia seeds

- 1 cup unsweetened almond milk (or other plant-based milk of choice)
- 1 teaspoon maple syrup or honey (optional for sweetness)
- Toppings: fresh berries, sliced bananas, chopped nuts, shredded coconut

Instructions:

- In a jar or bowl, mix together the chia seeds and almond milk.
- If desired, sweeten with honey or maple syrup.
- Refrigerate overnight or for at least 2 hours until the chia seeds have absorbed the liquid and the mixture has thickened.
- In the morning, give the chia pudding a good stir and add your favorite toppings.
- Enjoy this nutrient-rich and filling breakfast.

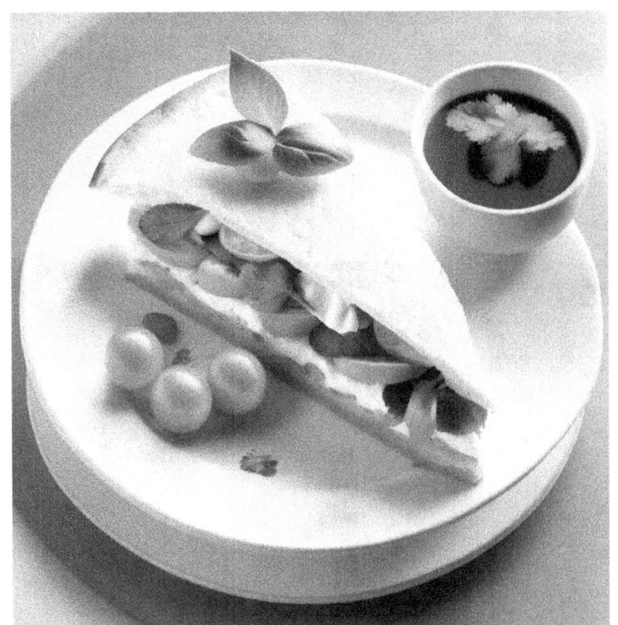

<u>Veggie Omelet</u>

Veggie Omelet:

Ingredients:

- 3 eggs (or egg whites)
- 1/4 cup diced bell peppers
- 1/4 cup diced onions
- Handful of spinach leaves
- Salt and pepper to taste
- 1 tsp olive oil (for cooking)

Instructions:

- Salt and pepper should be added to the eggs as you whisk them. In a mixing basin.
- Over medium heat, heat the olive oil in a nonstick skillet.
- Add the bell peppers and onions and sauté until softened.
- Spinach leaves should be added and cooked until wilted.
- Pour the whisked eggs into the skillet, tilting it to spread the mixture evenly.
- Cook for a few minutes until the eggs are set, then carefully flip the omelet and cook for another minute.
- The omelet should be folded in half after being slid onto a plate. Serve with a side of whole-grain toast or fresh fruit for a complete and satisfying breakfast.

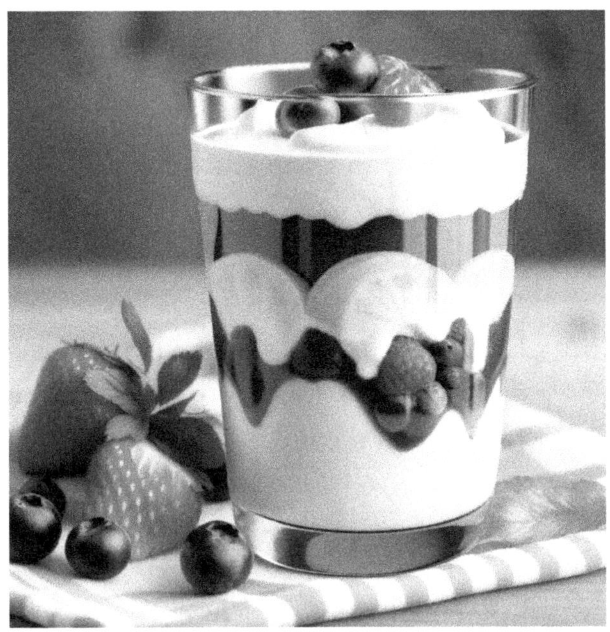

Greek Yogurt Parfait

Greek Yogurt Parfait:

Ingredients:

- 1 cup Greek yogurt (plain or flavored)
- 1/4 cup granola (look for low-sugar options or make your own)
- Handful of mixed berries (such as blueberries, strawberries, and raspberries)
- 1 tbsp honey or maple syrup (optional for extra sweetness)

Instructions:

- Layer Greek yogurt, granola, and mixed berries in a glass or bowl.
- Drizzle with maple syrup or honey if preferred.
- The layers should be repeated until all the ingredients are used
- Enjoy this protein-packed and nutrient-dense breakfast that provides a balance of flavors and textures.

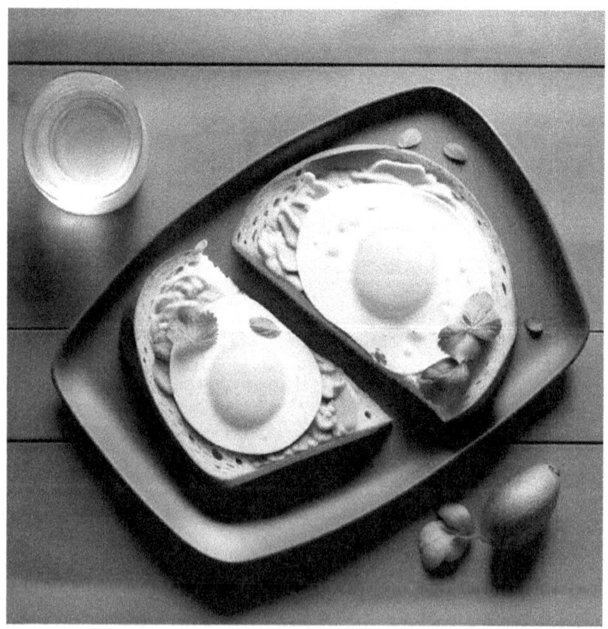

<u>Avocado Toast with Egg</u>

Ingredients:

- 1 slice of whole-grain bread (toasted)
- 1/2 ripe avocado, mashed
- 1 boiled or poached egg
- A sprinkle of red pepper flakes (optional)
- Salt and pepper to taste

Instructions:

- Evenly spread the mashed avocado on the toasted bread.
- Place the boiled or poached egg on top of the avocado.
- Sprinkle with red pepper flakes, salt, and pepper.
- Enjoy this simple and nutritious breakfast that provides healthy fats, protein, and fiber.

Feel free to customize these breakfast ideas with your favorite ingredients and flavors. Remember to listen to your body's needs and choose options that provide a good balance of nutrients to start your day off right!

Here are some satisfying lunch and dinner ideas that you can enjoy as part of your anti-inflammatory diet:

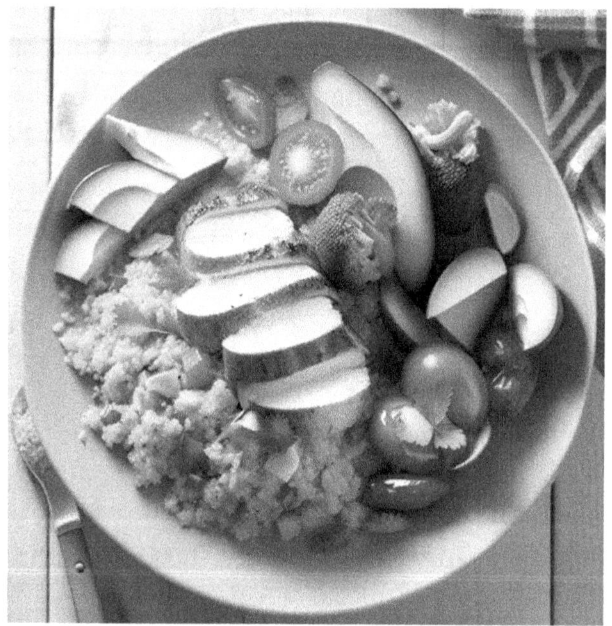

Quinoa Salad with Grilled Chicken and Avocado

Lunch: Quinoa Salad with Grilled Chicken and Avocado:

Ingredients:
- 1 cup cooked quinoa
- Grilled chicken breast, sliced

- 1/4 cup diced cucumber
- 1/4 cup cherry tomatoes, halved
- 1/4 cup diced red onion
- 1/4 cup sliced avocado
- A handful of mixed greens
- Lemon vinaigrette dressing (lemon juice, olive oil, Dijon mustard, salt, and pepper)

Instructions:

- In a bowl, combine the cooked quinoa, grilled chicken, cucumber, cherry tomatoes, red onion, avocado, and mixed greens.
- Drizzle with the lemon vinaigrette dressing and toss to combine.
- Adjust the seasoning if needed.
- Enjoy this protein-packed and fiber-rich salad for a satisfying and nourishing lunch.

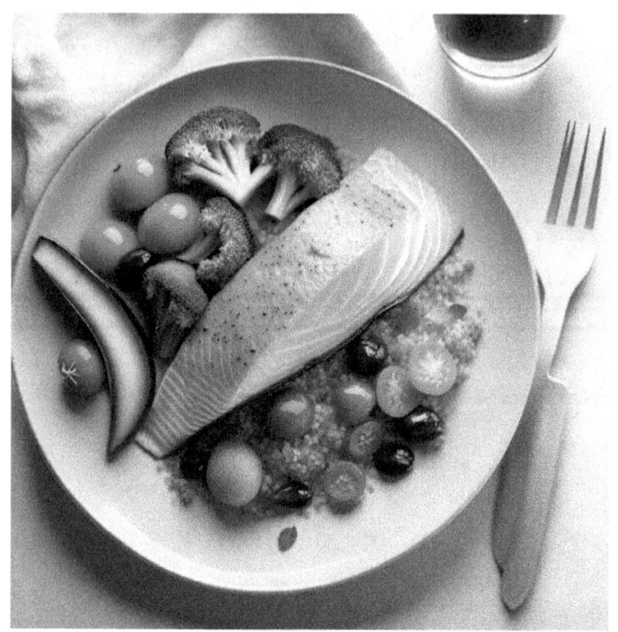

<u>Baked Salmon with Roasted Vegetables and Quinoa</u>

Dinner: Baked Salmon with Roasted Vegetables and Quinoa:

Ingredients:

- Salmon fillet
- Assorted vegetables (such as broccoli, cauliflower, carrots, and bell peppers), cut into bite-sized pieces
- Olive oil
- Lemon juice

- Salt and pepper
- Cooked quinoa

Instructions:
- Preheat the oven to 400°F (200°C).
- Place the salmon fillet on a baking sheet lined with parchment paper.
- Season with salt and pepper and drizzle with olive oil and lemon juice.
- In a separate baking dish, toss the vegetables with olive oil, salt, and pepper.
- Bake the salmon and vegetables in the oven for about 15-20 minutes, or until the salmon is cooked through and the vegetables are tender.
- Serve the baked salmon and roasted vegetables with a side of cooked quinoa.
- This flavorful and nutritious meal is rich in omega-3 fatty acids, vitamins, and antioxidants.

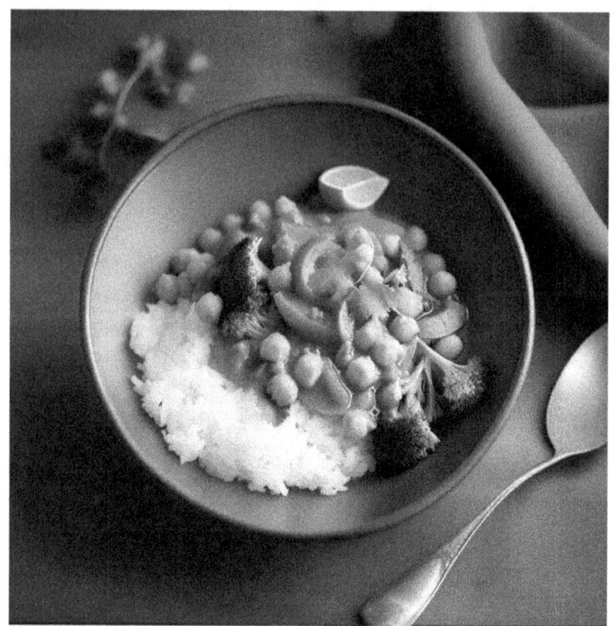

Chickpea and Vegetable Curry

Lunch or Dinner: Chickpea and Vegetable Curry:

Ingredients:

- 1 can chickpeas, drained and rinsed
- Assorted vegetables (such as bell peppers, zucchini, cauliflower, and carrots), diced
- 1 onion, diced
- 2 cloves garlic, minced
- 1 tsp grated ginger
- 1 can of coconut milk

- 2 tbsp curry powder
- 1 tsp turmeric powder
- Salt and pepper to taste
- Fresh cilantro (optional, for garnish)
- Cooked brown rice or quinoa

Instructions:

- In a large pot, sauté the onion, garlic, and ginger until fragrant.
- Add the diced vegetables and cook until slightly softened.
- Stir in the curry powder and turmeric powder, and cook for another minute.
- Add the chickpeas and coconut milk, and season with salt and pepper.
- Simmer the curry for about 15-20 minutes, or until the vegetables are cooked to your liking.
- Serve the chickpea and vegetable curry over cooked brown rice or quinoa.
- Garnish with fresh cilantro if desired.
- Enjoy this hearty and flavorful curry that is packed with plant-based protein and fiber.

Remember to adjust the portion sizes and ingredients based on your individual needs and preferences. These meals provide a good balance of nutrients and flavors, making them satisfying and nourishing.

Delicious Snacks and Desserts

Here are some delicious snack and dessert ideas that are also in line with an anti-inflammatory diet:

Snacks:

- **Greek Yogurt with Berries and Almonds**

Spoonfuls of Greek yogurt topped with a handful of fresh berries (such as strawberries, blueberries, and raspberries) and a sprinkle of sliced almonds.

- **Carrot Sticks with Hummus**

Enjoy raw carrot sticks dipped in a serving of homemade hummus, which can be made by blending cooked chickpeas, tahini, lemon juice, garlic, and olive oil.

- **Apple Slices with Almond Butter**

Slice a fresh apple and serve it with a side of almond butter for a satisfying combination of crispness and creaminess.

- **Mixed Nuts and Seeds**

Create a custom mix of your favorite nuts and seeds, such as almonds, walnuts, pumpkin seeds, and sunflower seeds, for a crunchy and nutrient-dense snack.

Desserts:

- **Berry Parfait**

Layer mixed berries (strawberries, blueberries, and raspberries) with a dollop of Greek yogurt and a sprinkle of granola or crushed nuts for a refreshing and nutritious dessert.

- **Chocolate Avocado Mousse**

Blend ripe avocados, cocoa powder, a touch of honey or maple syrup, and a splash of almond milk to create a rich and creamy chocolate mousse with a healthy twist.

- **Baked Apples with Cinnamon**

Core an apple, sprinkle it with cinnamon, and bake until tender. Enjoy it warm, and for extra indulgence, top it with a spoonful of Greek yogurt or a drizzle of honey.

- **Chia Seed Pudding**

Combine chia seeds with your choice of plant-based milk (such as almond milk or coconut milk) and a natural sweetener (such as honey or maple syrup). Let it sit in the refrigerator overnight, and in the morning, you'll have a delightful and nutritious pudding-like dessert.

Remember to enjoy these snacks and desserts in moderation while paying attention to portion sizes. They provide a balance of flavors and textures while incorporating anti-inflammatory ingredients to satisfy your cravings.

Chapter 5

Beyond Food: Additional Anti-Inflammatory Strategies

In addition to following an anti-inflammatory diet, there are several other strategies you can incorporate into your lifestyle to further reduce inflammation and promote overall well-being.

Here are some additional anti-inflammatory strategies:

- **Regular Exercise**

Exercise regularly, whether it be cycling, swimming, walking, or jogging. Exercise helps reduce inflammation and promotes the release of endorphins, which are natural mood-boosting chemicals in the body.

- **Stress Management**

Practice stress-reducing techniques like deep breathing exercises, meditation, yoga, or mindfulness. Chronic stress can contribute to inflammation, so finding healthy ways to manage stress is important.

- **Quality Sleep**

Prioritize getting enough sleep each night. Aim for 7-9 hours of uninterrupted sleep. Poor sleep can lead to increased inflammation, so establishing a regular sleep routine and creating a relaxing sleep environment are crucial.

- **Hydration**

To stay hydrated, drink a lot of water throughout the day. Water helps flush out toxins from the body and supports overall health. Aim for at least 8 cups (64 ounces) of water daily, or more depending on your activity level and individual needs.

- **Mindful Eating**

To practice mindful eating, pay attention to your body's hunger and fullness cues. Eat slowly, savoring each bite, and listen to your body's signals of satisfaction. This promotes healthy digestion and helps to prevent overeating.

- **Herbal Teas**

Incorporate anti-inflammatory herbal teas into your daily routine, such as turmeric tea, ginger tea, green tea, or chamomile tea. These teas contain compounds that have anti-inflammatory properties and can help soothe the body.

- **Adequate Omega-3 Fatty Acids**

Include foods rich in omega-3 fatty acids in your diet, such as fatty fish (salmon, mackerel, sardines), chia seeds, flaxseeds, and walnuts. Omega-3 fatty acids have anti-inflammatory effects and can support overall health.

- **Limit Alcohol and Tobacco**

Reduce or eliminate alcohol consumption and avoid tobacco products. Both alcohol and tobacco can promote inflammation in the body and have negative effects on overall health.

- **Maintain a Healthy Weight**

Try to maintain a healthy weight with a well-balanced diet and regular exercise. Excess body weight can contribute to chronic inflammation, so achieving and maintaining a healthy weight is beneficial.

- **Seek Professional Guidance**

If you have specific health concerns or conditions, consult with a healthcare professional or a registered dietitian for personalized advice and guidance on managing inflammation through diet and lifestyle.

By incorporating these strategies into your daily routine, you can further support your anti-inflammatory efforts and enhance your overall well-being.

Exercise and Movement

Exercise and movement play a crucial role in promoting overall health and reducing inflammation.

Consider the following key points:

- **Aerobic Exercise**

Engage in aerobic activities that increase your heart rate and breathing, such as walking, jogging, cycling, swimming, or dancing. Aim for at least 150 minutes of moderate-intensity aerobic exercise or 75 minutes of vigorous-intensity exercise per week, or a combination of both.

- **Strength Training**

Incorporate strength training exercises into your routine at least two days a week. Weightlifting, bodyweight exercises, and resistance band workouts are examples of such activities. Strength training helps build muscle mass, improve bone density, and support joint health.

- **Flexibility and Stretching**

Include stretching exercises to improve flexibility and mobility. Yoga, Pilates, and dedicated stretching routines can help enhance muscle flexibility, reduce muscle tension, and improve overall posture and movement.

- **Low-Impact Exercises**

If you have joint issues or limitations, consider low-impact exercises that are gentler on the joints. Options include swimming, water aerobics, elliptical training, or using a stationary bike. These activities can provide cardiovascular benefits without excessive stress on the joints.

- **Interval Training**

Consider incorporating interval training into your workouts. This includes alternating periods of high-intensity exercise with periods of lower intensity or rest. Interval training can be an effective way to improve cardiovascular fitness and burn calories.

- **Active Lifestyle**

Try to increase your everyday activity by finding opportunities to move more. Take the stairs instead of the elevator, walk or bike for short errands, or schedule active breaks throughout your workday. Find activities that you enjoy and incorporate them into your everyday routine.

- **Listen to Your Body**

Pay attention to your body's cues and adjust the intensity and duration of your workouts accordingly. It's important to challenge yourself, but also to respect your limits and avoid overexertion or injury. Increase the intensity and duration of your workouts gradually over time.

- **Stay Consistent**

Consistency is key when it comes to exercise. Aim for regular, balanced exercise throughout the week rather than sporadic intense workouts. Find a schedule that works for you and make exercise a part of your lifestyle.

Before starting any new exercise program always remember to consult with a healthcare professional, especially if you have any underlying health conditions or concerns. Based on your specific requirements and objectives, they may offer tailored advice.

Stress Reduction and Mindfulness

Stress reduction and mindfulness techniques are powerful tools for promoting overall well-being and reducing inflammation.

Here are some strategies to incorporate into your daily life:

- **Mindful Breathing**

Take a few moments during the day to focus on your breath. Deep, slow breaths can aid in the activation of the body's relaxation response and reduce stress. To practice diaphragmatic breathing, inhale deeply through your nose, allowing your abdomen to expand, and exhale slowly through your mouth.

- **Meditation**

Each day, set aside dedicated time for meditation. Find a quiet and comfortable space, close your eyes, and focus on your breath, a specific word or phrase (mantra), or an object. Meditation helps calm the mind, reduce stress, and promote mental clarity and emotional balance.

- **Mindful Eating**

Pay attention to the sensory experience of eating to practice mindful eating. Slow down, savor each bite, and observe the flavors, textures, and smells of your food. Pay attention to your body's hunger and fullness cues, and eat without distractions to fully engage in the present moment.

- **Nature Walks or Outdoor Time**

Spend time in nature to promote relaxation and reduce stress. Take walks in natural surroundings, go for hikes, or simply sit in a park. Connect with the sights, sounds, and sensations of the natural world around you to help calm your mind and find tranquility.

- **Gratitude Practice**

Focus on the positive aspects of your life to cultivate an attitude of gratitude. Take time each day to think about what you are grateful for. This practice can shift your perspective, enhance feelings of contentment, and reduce stress.

- **Mindful Movement**

Engage in activities that promote mindful movements, such as yoga, Tai Chi, or Qigong. These practices combine physical movement with breath awareness and mental focus, promoting relaxation, flexibility, and mind-body connection.

- **Digital Detox**

Take regular breaks from technology and social media. Set aside specific times each day to disconnect from screens and engage in activities that promote relaxation and self-care, such as reading, journaling, or spending quality time with loved ones.

- **Prioritize Self-Care**

Try to relax and have fun by doing things you enjoy. This can include hobbies, creative pursuits, spending time with loved ones, taking baths, practicing self-care rituals, or engaging in activities that promote relaxation and rejuvenation.

- **Seek Support**

Reach out to friends, family, or a support network when you need to talk or share your feelings. Sometimes, simply expressing your thoughts and emotions can help alleviate stress. Consider seeking professional help from a therapist or counselor if you're struggling with chronic stress or anxiety.

- **Establish Healthy Boundaries**

Learn to set boundaries and prioritize your well-being. Say no to activities or commitments that overwhelm you and learn to delegate tasks when possible. Recognize your limits and give yourself permission to take care of yourself first.

Remember, reducing stress and practicing mindfulness is a journey, so be patient with yourself. Incorporate these strategies gradually into your daily routine, and over time, you'll cultivate a greater sense of calm, resilience, and well-being.

Supplements and Lifestyle Changes

In addition to following an anti-inflammatory diet and incorporating stress reduction techniques, there are some supplements and lifestyle changes that can further support your overall well-being and reduce inflammation.

Here are a few to consider:

- **Omega-3 Fatty Acids**

Omega-3 fatty acids, found in fish oil supplements or derived from plant-based sources like flaxseed or chia seeds, have anti-inflammatory properties. Consider incorporating omega-3 supplements into your routine, but consult with a healthcare professional to determine the appropriate dosage for your specific needs.

- **Probiotics**

Probiotics are helpful bacteria that support a healthy gut microbiome. They can help in the reduction of inflammation and the improvement of gut health. Look for a high-quality probiotic supplement or incorporate probiotic-rich foods like yogurt, kefir, sauerkraut, or kimchi into your diet.

- **Vitamin D**

Vitamin D plays a role in modulating inflammation and supporting immune function. Depending on your geographic location and sun exposure, you may consider a vitamin D supplement. However, it's best to have your vitamin D levels checked and consult with a healthcare professional for personalized guidance.

- **Curcumin**

Curcumin is the active compound found in turmeric, known for its anti-inflammatory properties. Consider taking a curcumin supplement, but ensure it contains piperine (black pepper extract) to enhance absorption. Alternatively, you can incorporate turmeric into your cooking or enjoy turmeric tea.

- **Exercise Regularly**

Regular physical activity supports overall health and reduces inflammation. Aim for a mix of cardiovascular, strength training, and flexibility exercises. Find activities you enjoy doing and include them in your daily routine.

- **Quality Sleep**

Prioritize getting enough sleep each night. Create a calming bedtime routine, ensure your sleep environment is comfortable and dark, and avoid electronic devices before bed. Quality sleep supports overall well-being and helps regulate inflammation in the body.

- **Stress Management**

Chronic stress can contribute to inflammation, so it's important to incorporate stress management techniques. Relaxation practices such as meditation, deep breathing, and yoga can help. Engage in activities that bring you joy, and consider seeking support from a therapist or counselor if needed.

- **Smoking Cessation**

If you smoke, consider quitting. Smoking is a major contributor to inflammation and numerous health issues. Seek support from support groups, healthcare professionals, or smoking cessation programs to help you quit successfully.

- **Hydration**

Drink plenty of water throughout the day to stay hydrated. Water helps flush out toxins, supports digestion, and promotes overall health. Aim for at least 8 cups (64 ounces) of water daily, or more depending on your activity level and individual needs.

- **Mindfulness and Relaxation**

Incorporate mindfulness and relaxation practices into your daily life. Engage in activities that promote relaxation, such as reading, listening to calming music, taking baths, or spending time in nature. Find moments to disconnect and rejuvenate.

Remember, it's important to consult with a healthcare professional before starting any new supplements, especially if you have underlying health conditions or are taking medications. They can provide personalized advice and guidance based on your individual needs and help ensure the supplements are safe and appropriate for you.

Conclusion

In conclusion, adopting an anti-inflammatory diet and incorporating lifestyle changes can have a profound impact on your overall health and well-being. By understanding the role of food in the inflammatory process and making informed choices, you can unleash the power of the anti-inflammatory diet to nourish your body and flourish in life.

Throughout this book, we explored the basics of inflammation and how it relates to the foods we consume. We delved into the benefits of an anti-inflammatory diet, identifying the foods that promote inflammation and those that help combat it. We learned about the power of plant-based foods, healthy fats, and proteins in reducing inflammation and supporting optimal health.

We discussed the importance of herbs, spices, and other natural ingredients that possess anti-inflammatory properties, allowing us to enhance the flavor of our meals while also promoting wellness. We also explored the foods to avoid and the hidden inflammatory culprits that may be hindering our progress.

To help you put theory into practice, we provided a comprehensive anti-inflammatory meal plan, including a 7-day meal plan with delicious and nutritious recipes to fuel your day from breakfast to dinner. We also shared meal planning tips and tricks to simplify the process and make it more enjoyable.

However, we went beyond food alone. We recognized the importance of other lifestyle factors in reducing inflammation and promoting overall well-being. We explored the significance of exercise and movement, stress reduction techniques, and the practice of mindfulness. Additionally, we discussed the role of supplements and highlighted the importance of quality sleep, hydration, and other lifestyle changes.

By embracing these recommendations, you can unlock the full potential of the anti-inflammatory diet and transform your health from the inside out. Remember, every small step you take towards reducing inflammation and prioritizing your well-being is a step towards nourishing your body and allowing it to flourish.

Ultimately, the journey towards an anti-inflammatory lifestyle is a lifelong commitment. It requires mindfulness, patience, and self-compassion. Embrace the power of the anti-inflammatory diet, make choices that support your well-being, and enjoy the countless benefits that come from nourishing your body and unleashing its true potential. Here's to a life filled with vitality, health, and flourishing!

Embracing the Anti-Inflammatory Lifestyle

Embracing the anti-inflammatory lifestyle is a transformative journey that goes beyond just following a diet plan. It involves making conscious choices that prioritize your health and well-being.

Here are some key points to keep in mind as you embrace this lifestyle:

- **Mindful Eating**

Practice mindful eating by being fully present and aware of the foods you consume. Pay attention to your body's hunger and fullness cues, and choose nutrient-dense, whole foods that nourish your body and support inflammation reduction.

• Meal Planning and Preparation

Plan your meals in advance and prepare homemade meals as much as possible. This allows you to have better control over the ingredients you use and ensures that you have nourishing options readily available.

• Emphasize Plant-Based Foods

Incorporate a wide variety of colorful fruits, vegetables, whole grains, legumes, nuts, and seeds into your meals. These plant-based foods are rich in antioxidants, fiber, and other essential nutrients that promote overall health and fight inflammation.

• Healthy Fats and Proteins

Include healthy fats like avocados, olive oil, and nuts, as well as lean proteins such as fish, poultry, tofu, and beans in your diet. This help provides essential nutrients and supports a balanced anti-inflammatory approach.

• Minimize Processed Foods

Reduce your consumption of processed and packaged foods that often contain artificial additives, preservatives, and unhealthy fats. Whenever possible, choose whole, unprocessed foods.

- **Stay Hydrated**

Drink plenty of water throughout the day to support hydration and proper bodily functions. Water helps flush out toxins and aids in maintaining overall health.

- **Regular Physical Activity**

Engage in regular exercise and movement to promote circulation, reduce inflammation, and support overall well-being. Find activities you enjoy doing and include them in your daily routine.

- **Stress Reduction**

Manage stress through practices such as meditation, deep breathing, yoga, or engaging in hobbies that bring you joy. Chronic stress can contribute to inflammation, so finding healthy ways to manage it is crucial.

- **Quality Sleep**

Prioritize quality sleep by establishing a consistent sleep routine, creating a comfortable sleep environment, and practicing relaxation techniques before bed. Restorative sleep helps support your body's natural healing processes.

- **Seek Support and Accountability**

Find an accountability partner who shares your goals or surround yourself with a supportive community. Having someone to share your challenges, successes, and progress with can help keep you motivated and on track.

Remember, embracing the anti-inflammatory lifestyle is a lifelong commitment. It's not about perfection, but rather about making consistent, mindful choices that support your health and well-being. Celebrate your progress, be kind to yourself, and enjoy the positive impact that the anti-inflammatory lifestyle can have on your overall quality of life.

Continuing Your Journey to Optimal Health

Congratulations on taking the first steps towards embracing an anti-inflammatory lifestyle! As you continue on your journey to optimal health, here are some key points to keep in mind:

- **Regular Check-Ins**

To assess your progress and make any necessary adjustments, schedule regular check-ins with yourself. Listen to your body and pay attention to how certain foods, activities, or lifestyle choices make you feel. This self-awareness will guide you in making informed decisions that best support your well-being.

- **Personalize Your Approach**

Everyone's body is unique, so it's important to personalize your approach to the anti-inflammatory lifestyle. Experiment with different foods, recipes, and strategies to find what works best for you. Consider working with a healthcare professional or registered dietitian who can provide personalized guidance based on your specific needs and goals.

- **Stay Informed**

Continue to educate yourself about the latest research and information related to inflammation and health. Stay up-to-date with reputable sources and be open to new insights that can enhance your understanding and guide your choices.

• Practice Mindful Indulgence

It's important to strike a balance between nourishing your body and enjoying the pleasures of life. Allow yourself occasional indulgences, such as a small treat or a meal that may not align perfectly with the anti-inflammatory guidelines. Practice mindfulness and savor these moments, but always come back to your commitment to nourishing your body and reducing inflammation.

• Support Gut Health

The health of your gut plays a crucial role in inflammation and overall well-being. Support your gut health by incorporating probiotic-rich foods, such as fermented vegetables and yogurt, and prebiotic foods, such as onions, garlic, and whole grains, into your diet. Consider adding a high-quality probiotic supplement if needed.

• Adjust as Needed

As your body changes and evolves, so too might your nutritional and lifestyle needs. Be willing to adjust along the way. Periodically reassess your goals and make any necessary modifications to your diet, exercise routine, stress management techniques, or supplements to ensure they continue to support your optimal health.

- **Share Your Knowledge**

Share your knowledge and experiences with others who may benefit from an anti-inflammatory lifestyle. Inspire and support those around you by sharing healthy recipes, tips, and information. By fostering a community of wellness, you can make a positive impact on others' lives.

- **Celebrate Progress**

No matter how small, celebrate your achievements and milestones. Acknowledge the positive changes you've made and the impact they have on your health. Cultivate a mindset of gratitude and self-compassion, recognizing that this journey is about progress, not perfection.

Remember, your journey to optimal health is a lifelong commitment. It's about making sustainable changes that support your well-being and nourish your body from the inside out. Embrace the journey with an open mind, be kind to yourself, and enjoy the abundant benefits that come from living an anti-inflammatory lifestyle. Here's to your continued growth, vitality, and optimal health!